Celery Juic

I0037417

The Complete Recipe Guide for Staying Healthy

Kevin Mary Neo

Table of Contents

Copyright © 2021 by Kevin Mary Neo

All rights reserved. No part of this publication may be reproduced, distributed, or transmitted in any form or by any means, including photocopying, recording, or other electronic or mechanical methods, without the prior written permission of the publisher, except in the case of brief quotations embodied in critical reviews and certain other non-commercial uses permitted by copyright law.

ISBN: 978-1-63750-107-8

Introduction

The celery juice movement demands to drink blended and drained celery each morning on a clear stomach to be able to "produce sweeping improvements for all sorts of medical issues." Some celebrity testimonials promoting the drink made the celery juice hype spread across social networking.

This sad news implies that registered dietitians, food scientists, and biochemists are mourning the increased loss of another nutrient-dense food turned "cure-all" by a method practiced and supported by some A-list celebrity.

What's celery juice?

Celery juice is made by blending and straining celery. The entire stalks of celery pack a lot of minerals and vitamins, including vitamin K, vitamin A, potassium, and folate; but from a nutrition standpoint, celery juice takes phytonutrient-filled produce and turns it right into a concentrated way to obtain sugar. In most cases, no matter how much or how little sugar a vegetable or fruit contains, juicing it will yield an increased concentration of sugar per fluid ounce than you'll take in grams.

Does celery juice assist with chronic inflammation?

The Medical Medium blog claims that celery juice is teeming with powerful anti-inflammatory properties. Celery is ideal for reversing inflammation since it starves the pathogens, such as, unproductive bacteria and viruses. Celery deprives isease-causing pathogens of fuel.

Celery Juice can cure all sorts of illnesses. Scientific data actually shows that celery juice contains antioxidant compounds called flavones. It's biochemically plausible that flavones could stop specific reactions within you that result in chronic inflammation, subsequently lowering your threat of chronic disease.

Information continues to be limited on how bioavailable (actually usable), these compounds are in humans. Most research up to now continues to be performed on lab rats or in test tubes, however, despite its possibility, it doesn't make it entirely applicable for an everyday life. Most of us own completely different, unique lifestyles that affect our body's cells. Producing the jump from potential advantages to highly good for people who have problems with chronic and mystery illnesses isn't just a jump, it's an abuse of existing data. It's actively not considering what else we may eat per day, week, or year.

Chapter 1

Celery

Celery, also called *Apium graveolens* is a marshland plant from the family *Apiaceae* that is cultivated all over the world for a long period. Celery includes a lengthy fibrous stalk that tapers into leaves. This plant is currently an integral part of the American, Irish, Japanese and Australian cuisines. It is most commonly found in soups and salads or as a garnish to dishes. Additionally, it is consumed as a snack since it is fairly filling.

Vitamins and Minerals Composition of Celery

Celery is abundant with Vitamin K and Molybdenum. In addition, it contains folate, potassium, soluble fiber, manganese, and pantothenic acid. Aside from these, celery also includes Vitamin B_2, copper, Vitamin C, vitamin B_6, Calcium, Phosphorus, Magnesium and Vitamin A.

Health Advantages of Celery

Aids in preventing cancer

Phthalides, flavonoids, and polyacetylenes, that have cancer-fighting houses, can be found in celery. They help detoxify the carcinogens. Celery also includes coumarins that improve the actions of particular white blood cells and may effectively fight cancer as well. These components have a tendency to act against free radicals floating inside our body and neutralize them before they are able to cause any harm.

Help reduce blood circulation pressure

Phthalides, organic compounds within celery, help reduce the degree of stress hormones within your blood. This can help your arteries to expand and facilitates the smooth blood circulation and, thus, reduces blood circulation pressure. When blood circulation pressure is usually reduced, the probability of developing atherosclerosis, coronary attack or heart stroke also drops.

Aids in preventing ulcers

Celery contains a particular kind of ethanol extract that's useful in protecting the lining of the digestive system from ulcers. Celery extract has the capacity to replenish depleted degrees of gastric mucus that's needed within the stomach lining to avoid the forming of microscopic holes and openings. Additionally, it is thought that celery nourishes the stomach, colon, and intestines because of the existence of chemical constituents like flavonoids, tannins, volatile oils and alkaloids.

Checks urinary system infection

Celery seeds are known and used because of its diuretic properties, since it assists with the elimination of the crystals. Uric acid is usually excreted via urination. Consequently, people who have bladder disorders, kidney problems, cystitis along with other similar problems will see its good if celery seeds are within their diet. These seeds are also be best for women experiencing urinary system infection.

Detoxifies the body

All elements of the celery plant including seeds, roots, and leaves could be used as antioxidants. You are able to avoid diseases from the kidney, pancreas, liver, and gallbladder by incorporating this vegetable in what you eat.

Helps to strengthen immunity

Celery seeds have certain anti-microbial effects which allow it to be utilized like a herbal medicine for years over years. When extracts from celery seeds are blended with parasites compounds that cause infection in humans, the extract could purify and decrease bacteria's growth. This shows that celery can enhance your immunity and fight transmissions.

Fix for arthritis

Celery offers anti-inflammatory properties that helps reduce swelling and pain around the joints. This makes it good for people who have arthritis, rheumatism and gout. It help remove uric acid crystals from your own body and enable you to get rest from joint pain. In addition, it helps to raise the regrowth of tissue in inflamed joints.

Really helps to control diabetes

Celery leaves possess a high content material of fiber and really which helps to manage diabetes. Celery works well in fighting Type-2 diabetes.

Really helps to reduce weight

Celery has very less calories and it is quite filling since it is abundant with fiber. This makes it ideal to truly have a glass of celery juice before meals so you look full and don't overeat. This will bring your bodyweight down and in addition will not make you to feel hunger on a regular basis.

Prevents Cataracts

Cataracts is an illness that results in a partial lack of vision and generally afflicts the Elderly. Dripping celery tea drops on eyelids is wonderful for certain ophthalmological circumstances and can increase your eye health, reduces the probability of your eyes getting cataracts as well as prevents macular degeneration.

Brings relief from migraine

Celery contains coumarins that may provide rest from migraines. Research indicates that coumarins help suppress the discharge of nitric oxide in the mind, which may cause headaches and migraines.

Uses of Celery

Celery really helps to manage diabetic symptoms, gives rest from asthma and migraine, promotes cardiovascular health insurance and also prevents the onset of cancer. In addition, it helps to reduce blood circulation pressure and blood cholesterol, prevents urinary system infections in females, it also helps to reduce swelling and pain across the joints and improves eye health.

Side-Effects & Allergies of Celery

Despite all its beneficial effects, celery belongs to a little band of foods that could cause a severe allergic attack in a few people which might trigger a fatal anaphylactic shock. Celery can be bad for women that are pregnant as its seeds contain volatile oils, flavonoids, coumarins and linoleic acid that could cause contractions inside the uterus.

Cultivation of Celery

The uses of celery could be traced back again to ancient times and records which show that celery leaves were found in the area within the tomb of Pharaoh King Tutankhamen who died in 1323 B.C. In ancient Greece, celery leaves were used as garlands for the dead also to produce wreaths and garlands for the victors in battle. Now it's a part of cuisines all around the globe. A big part of Punjab develops celery for export into Europe, where it is used as a condiment.

Celery grows best where the winters are cold as well as the summers are hot since it is a cool weather crop. The celery seeds are small plus they ought to be covered lightly with soil and watered evenly for 3-8 weeks or started indoors and transferred outside after 2 months.

Undesirable Effects of Celery

Celery scientific brand *Apium graveolens* is actually a plant whose crisp green stalks are eaten both raw and cooked. Native towards the Mediterranean region, it has been cultivated since ancient greek times. Celery is definitely a common element of weight-loss diets, as it's lower in calories and saturated in nutrients. Celery seed can be sometimes used as an herbal remedy. There are a few health issues regarding celery which every consumer of celery juice ought to be familiar with.

Allergic Reactions

Celery is an extremely common allergen and reactions to it could be life-threatening. If you are allergic to birch pollen or mugwort, you're also more likely to respond to celery. Symptoms range from itching and rashes, swelling of the facial skin, mouth, tongue, and throat, dizziness to stomach upset. A far more severe reaction called anaphylactic shock is marked by lightheadedness, a drop in blood pressure, rapid pulse and difficulty in breathing. Anaphylactic shock can be a serious medical problem that can result in coma and death. Cooking will not affect the allergenic potential of celery.

Photosensitivity

Celery contains many compounds referred to as furanocoumarins. These chemicals cause the skin to become photosensitive, in that, they become sensitive to bright light, especially sunlight. Usually, this reaction happens because of intensive handling; it's common amongst agricultural workers, for instance. However, Dermanet New Zealand reports that "occasionally, ingestion of the chemicals in celery soup could cause generalized sun sensitivity; several people have developed severe sunburn after eating celery soup and venturing out in sunlight or even to a tanning salon."

Kidney Issues

Celery is both abundant with water and an all-natural diuretic. So, people who have kidney problems should monitor their celery intake, as excessive consumption might put extra strain on the kidneys. Consult a doctor if that is a problem of yours.

Concerns for Women That Are Pregnant

Women that are pregnant should avoid large doses of celery and celery seed as it could induce bleeding and uterine contractions. Occasional consumption within a well-balanced diet isn't an issue.

How to Roast Celery

Celery got its reputation as the perfect diet food because of its low-calorie content. A single cup of raw celery has just 16 calories. Additionally, it is cholesterol-free, contains only a trace amount of fat and includes a high concentration of essential nutrients like vitamin K, vitamin A, and fluoride. While celery is frequently consumed raw or as an addition to soups, casseroles or stir-fries, roasting celery at a higher temperature can intensify the vegetable's flavor and caramelize its natural sugars, giving it a slightly sweet taste.

Some great cooks roast celery like a side dish for meat, poultry or fish or as an ingredient in risotto or pasta.

Preparation
Step 1
Remove as much celery stalks from the complete vegetable's base as you intend to roast. Wash each thoroughly under cool, running water and pat dry with paper towels.

Step 2

Trim off the finish and leafy tops of every celery stalk with a sharp knife. Slice the trimmed celery into bite-sized chunks.

Step 3

Line a rimmed baking sheet with aluminum foil or cooking parchment. Place the celery onto the baking sheet, drizzle the vegetables with olive oil and sprinkle them with salt and pepper, if desired. Use your hands to toss the celery until they are coated with the oil and seasonings.

Step 4

Place the baking sheet into an oven pre-heated to 400 degrees Fahrenheit. Allow the celery to roast, using tongs or perhaps a pancake turner to stir and turn the pieces every ten minutes.

Step 5

Roast the celery to your desired degree of tenderness, typically between fifteen to thirty minutes. Take away the baking sheet through the oven and serve the celery hot, cold or at room temperature.

Things You Will Need

- A couple of fresh celery
- Paper towels
- Sharp knife
- Cutting board
- Aluminum foil or cooking parchment
- Olive oil
- Salt and pepper, optional
- Tongs or pancake turner

The very best celery stalks to utilize for roasting will be the outermost stalks on a couple of whole fresh celery. When the stalks own tough strings, make use of a vegetable peeler to eliminate them. Season roasted celery with lemon juice, vinegar or the selection of seasoning. Reserve the leafy tops of trimmed celery to use in salads or soups.

How to Bake Celery

Celery can be a crisp vegetable that has vitamins A and C. Calcium can be found within celery. It is in the same family as carrots, and it could be purchased at any moment of the entire year. A multitude of various kinds of celery is grown, but Pascal celery may be the most familiar type. Celery could be enjoyed raw or cooked. One method to cook celery would be to bake it inside the oven. Whenever choosing celery, search for celery that's actually in color, do not accept celery that's rubbery. Also, check the leaves to be sure these are green. Remove strings before baking celery.

Step 1
Place your oven to 350 degrees to preheat it.

Step 2
Separate the celery stalks and wash them under cold running water.

Step 3
Blot the stalks dry with paper towels.

Step 4

Take away the strings in the celery stalks by forcing the edge of the small knife beneath the celery strings and securing them between your knife plus the pad of your respective thumb. With a grip, pull the knife and the end of the celery strings toward you. Do not stop pulling until you reach the end of every string and totally take it off. Be sure you consider all the celery strings out which means that your cooked celery is simple to chew.

Step 5

Lay each celery stalk down on the cutting board. Slice the stalks into 2-inch pieces.

Step 6

Position the celery pieces within the large pan, along with 1/4 cup of water.

Step 7

Bring the drinking water to some boil, then decrease the heat, cover the pan and cook the celery for approximately 11 minutes.

Step 8

Pour the celery and drinking water into the colander to drain from the normal water.

Step 9

Place the celery inside the glass baking dish and add the mushroom soup. Usually do not add water to the soup. Stir with a big spoon to mix the ingredients.

Step 10

Position the celery within the oven to bake for thirty minutes. Do not cover the celery.

Step 11

Sprinkle the French fried onion rings together with the celery after thirty minutes, and then place the celery back the oven to bake for another ten minutes.

Things You Will Need

- 1/2 couple of celery stalks
- Paper towels
- A small, sharp knife
- Cutting board

- Huge pan with cover
- 1/4 cup water
- Colander
- 3/4 can of mushroom soup, 10.5 oz. size
- Significant glass baking dish
- Large spoon
- 1/2 cup smashed french fried onion rings

Add more French fried onion rings in the event that you desire more. Season the baked celery with black pepper, if you want the taste of black pepper.

Are Parsley and Celery exactly the same?

Celery and parsley are from a similar botanical family as carrots, parsnips, dill, fennel and a huge selection of other well known plants. Even though crisp, fibrous stalks that define an average head of celery don't bear much resemblance towards the abundant, aromatic green leaves of fresh parsley, both foods are closely related.

Celery

Americans are most acquainted with pascal celery, an extremely cultivated variety that's considerably less stringy than wild celery. Even though the plant's leafy green top is often discarded, celery leaves are edible and like parsley, quite flavorful. Celery is often a low-calorie way to obtain vitamin C, potassium and soluble fiber. You can eat it raw or incorporate it into cooked dishes.

Parsley

Fresh parsley is known as an herb, meaning it's generally used to check or flavor other foodstuffs. While its long, thin stalks are edible, the plant is valued because of its bright green leaves, that are lower in calories and abundant with vitamins A, C, K, and folate, as well as iron, potassium, and fiber. You can eat parsley either raw or add it to cooked dishes right before serving.

Considerations

Using its ultra-thin stalks filled with bright green leaves, you could easily mistake leaf celery, also known as Chinese celery or Nan Ling celery for flat-leaf, or Italian, parsley. Leaf celery is simply as flavorful as parsley, and you may consume it raw or very lightly cooked. Chinese celery, that is often obtainable in Asian markets, appears like a cross between traditional celery and flat-leaf parsley.

Chapter 2

Celery Nourishment Information

Crunchy raw celery sticks make a nutritious snack to greatly help manage your body weight. You'll receive essential minerals and vitamins from celery which are needed to maintain your general health and maintain your disease fighting capability at its best. Try dipping celery sticks in a handful of low-fat salad dressing, hummus or peanut butter for just a little spare flavor or add celery to soups, stews, and casseroles to improve the quantity and nutrient content.

Calories, Fat and Protein

Celery is really a low-calorie and fat-free food ideal for assisting you to lose or sustain your weight. It's composed of 95 percent water by weight. All of this fluid can make you full and satisfied without contributing many calories. From 2 medium stalks of celery about 8 inches long, you'll get just 12 calories and 0.2 grams of fat. Additionally, there is significantly less than 1 gram of protein per portion of celery.

Carbohydrates

Celery is actually a low carbohydrate food, which fits well right into a meal arrange for diabetes or low-carb diets. Eating celery won't impact your blood sugar levels much since it simply contains 3 total carbohydrates per portion. About 1.5 grams of the carbohydrate is soluble fiber, which is indigestible but necessary to your health. Fiber absorbs water and swells within your digestive tract to supply bulk and keep foods moving through the body. Eating an ample amount of dietary fiber can help regulate digestion, sustain your weight, lower cholesterol as well as prevent certain types of cancer.

Vitamins

Eating celery within a balanced diet can help you meet your daily requirement of vitamin K. A serving of celery provides 23 micrograms of vitamin K, which is 29 percent from the day-by-day value. Adequate intake of vitamin K helps to ensure your blood clots properly. According to MedlinePlus, vitamin K are likely to be involved in maintaining bone relative density while one ages. You'll receive 8 percent in the day-by-day value for vitamin A as well as the B vitamin folate as well. These nutrients are crucial for cell formation as well as for keeping your eye, skin and bone health; they could also prevent certain birth defects.

Minerals

You'll also get some good essential minerals from eating celery. A serving of celery provides 6.5 percent with the daily value for potassium and 3 percent on the daily value for calcium. Both calcium and potassium work as electrolytes, which maintain electrical impulses within you and help regulate fluid balance. Meeting your daily needs for potassium also helps maintain your heart health and maintains proper blood pressure. Calcium plays a component in forming strong bones and teeth and in addition to hormone regulation.

Do Celery Leaves Have Vitamins And Minerals?

Next time you get celery, save the leaves to consume alone or include into recipes. Celery leaves offer vitamins and minerals that can increase your health. Celery leaves produce a great choice for weight-loss diets because they're lower in calories and offer vitamins, minerals, fiber, and macronutrients.

Calories and Fat

A 100 gram serving of celery leaves, about 3.5 ounces, introduces 34.8 calories into the meal plan. In the event that you observe a 2,000 calorie diet, the number in these leaves compatible 1.7 percent of the total allowable calories in a 24-hour period. Additionally, you ingest 0.3 grams of fat. A lot of the fat in celery leaves derives from polyunsaturated fat, some sort of healthy fat that positively influences cholesterol amounts and may reduce the threat to the heart and helps to maintain a glowing and hydrated skin. Since I added celery juice to my day-to-day routine, I've noticed my skin is a lot smoother and softer as I love. Water and antioxidant content material from the juice can be the best for purifying the body and producing the skin we want, Only a heads up though, be ready for some major breakouts when you initially begin drinking regularly since it literally pulls all the poisons and shits out of the body. I really like it since it actually shows me that it's working. I definitely have struggled with less breakouts the more consistent I am. Celery juice is packed with vitamin A, B, C, K, niacin and folate, which are crucial for repairing skin damages as well as maintaining the fitness of the skin we have. These vitamins also assist in producing collagen!

Hair

The high amount of water and vitamin A within celery juice is excellent for our hair! Drinking water keeps our scalp hydrated and cures dandruff, while vitamin A provides nourishment towards the roots of hair strands and makes them healthy. Celery juice can be recognized to stimulate the growth in our hair and improve its texture and make it softer.

Anti-Cancer Properties

Celery juice offers cancer-fighting properties. There are always a ton of anti-cancer substances within the juice that assist in cancer prevention in several ways. For instance, the acetylenic content material in the juice prevents the tumor cells from growing as well as the phenolic acid content makes the hormone-like prostaglandins inactive.

Blood Pressure

Celery juice also helps control your blood circulation pressure. The 3-n-butylphthalide within celery juice diminishes the secretion of stress hormones and relaxes the muscles present around our arteries.

Chapter 3

How to make Celery Juice

Celery juice is in fact super easy to create. When you have a juicer, then you are actually a pro and may figure this out for yourself. You should drink 16 oz of celery juice first thing each day. You might not want to do this, but we believe it is best if taken on a clear stomach. If you opt to drink at another period, we would suggest doing this 10-15 minutes before meals because it is usually super filling and I discover that it is most effective before eating.

Ingredients

- 3-5 celery stalks (use organic)
- Water
- Lemon (for taste - you can include in apple, cucumber, etc

Instructions

Step 1: wash the celery stalks

Step 2: slice the celery stalks into 4-inch pieces

Step 3: put the celery for your blender

Step 4: bring 1 cup of water

Step 5: blend until completely smooth

Step 6: make use of a strainer and pour celery juice into a cup

Step 7: Add some lemon juice in the event that you don't just like the taste.

Celery leaves themselves have high degrees of vitamin A plus the stalks contain vitamin C, B6, B2. and B1. Thus, when blended right into a juice, celery offers an entire host of other benefits.

Benefits of Celery Juice

Restore Body acidity

Celery may be used to support keep up with the balance between alkaline and acid within you. Celery actively minimizes your body's acidity, rendering your body even more alkalescent, maintaining your pH amounts and get it balanced.

These vital minerals work to neutralize any extra acidity that you might be experiencing.

Decrease Blood Pressure

Do You have an high blood circulation pressure? Celery's sodium amounts help to sustain your lymph and blood liquidity, ensuring your blood doesn't become too thick. Abundant with iron, and A and C vitamins, celery may also help forestall strokes, eliminate plaque within your arteries, and ultimately decrease your blood pressure.

Assist In Preventing Cancer

Prevent cancer by drinking celery juice each day. The celery contains anti-cancer compounds. The nutrients in celery help to get rid of the free radicals within you that can easily cause cancer. Phenolic acids in celery help block prostaglandins that could otherwise encourage the growth of tumor cells. The soothing and healing ramifications of this juice also help treat symptoms of cancer treatment, like IBS, Crohn's disease, and inflammation from digestive issues.

Lower Cholesterol levels

Utilize this juice as an all-natural remedy to lessen cholesterol in the body. This juice contains a substance called 3-n-butylphthalide which includes a positive ffect with reducing cholesterol within the blood.

Prevent Constipation

This juice gets the potential to cure several digestive process disorders as celery contains fibers that are laxative. Thus, this juice is quite effective in relieving constipation. It can help to relax your nerves inside your bowels, rendering it easier to proceed.

Used as a Diuretic

It facilitates the flow of urine by drinking even more of the juice. The potassium and sodium in the celery are all-natural diuretic; this helps to modify your urine production and means that it is possible to secrete waste in an effective manner.

Prevent Inflammation

Celery contains luteolin, the potent flavonoid that functions as an antioxidant to calm inflammation. The celery's polyacetylene also really helps to provide rest from inflammation due to gout, degenerative osteoarthritis, respiratory diseases, and arthritis.

Both compounds in celery has an ideal natural treatment for inflammation.

Improve Kidney Function

Celery juice may be used to improve kidney function by averting calcification within your kidneys, bladder, and gallbladder. The celery works to equalize the pH level in the torso and neutralize the acidity. By eliminating calcium deposits from your own joints, the celery can help the body complete its detoxification process.

Support Your Nervous System

Keep the nervous system in balance by causing a habit of regularly consuming this juice. The vitamins and minerals in this juice help sustain your nervous system, rendering it one of the better natural treatments for anyone attempting to combat insomnia and similar issues.

Assist in Weight Loss

Looking for a far more effective weight reduction regimen? Begin drinking considerably more of the juice. As celery is definitely filled with nutrients and vitamins, it's the perfect way to satiate your cravings. Lower in calories, making a habit of eating more of the juice can help you shed more inches earlier than you think.

Detoxify Your Liver

Did you find out that you will be constantly be coping with recurrent viruses, fungi, bacteria, along with other waste? It's time to take care of your liver with some celery juice. The photo nutrients in the celery will flush out your liver and make sure it is functioning effectively since it works to detoxify the body.

Increase Your Sleep

The magnesium within celery juice is incredibly effective in calming your body. With a scarcity of magnesium, you might encounter issues sleeping as well as other health issues. Begin sleeping better with the addition of even more celery to your daily diet. Promote stress-free rest by boosting your magnesium intake when you have more celery.

Promote Healthy Skin

Are store-bought skin treatments no longer working for you? Begin caring for your skin layer using the nutrients within celery. Celery works to set your skin layer and improve elasticity. Higher in vitamins K, B, C, and A, celery is actually a superfood with regards to improving the fineness of your skin. Using its raw juice, you'll have the ability to begin toning your skin layer and appearance younger than ever before.

Eliminate Pimples and Acne

Tired of coping with pimples and acne scarring? Begin taking your skin backward in age by drinking more of the juice.

All the powerful nutrients in this vegetable work to carefully turn back the consequences of acne while attempting to get rid of the excess oils that may result in acne.

Reduce Wrinkles

Signs of aging like wrinkles may also be treated with this magic elixir of a juice. As celery contains a multitude of nourishing vitamins, regularly drinking this juice can lead to the wrinkle-free and softer skin you've been desiring.

Remove Dandruff

Hydrate your scalp with the energy of the juice. The presence of vitamin A inside the celery will treat your hair roots and strands. Ultimately, these nutrients will continue to work to eliminate dandruff and keep your scalp free and clear.

Prevent Hair Thinning and Greying

Is your hair aging faster than you? Is it beginning to drop even more strands than you ought to be? Utilize this juice to start out stimulating hair regrowth. Furthermore, to turning back the clock on hair thinning, you should use this juice to boost nice hair texture and decrease the amount of graying you experience.

Prevent Jaundice

While jaundice isn't a typical concern for many people at this point in time, drinking this juice might help reduce the threat of developing jaundice. Its antioxidative properties work to keep your blood clean to avoid the bile buildup leading to the condition.

Prevent Dehydration

Celery undoubtedly contains a substantial amount of water. Consuming this vegetable helps to prevent dehydration.

Fight Bronchitis

In the event that you blend the complete celery stalk using the seeds and everything as you try to make the juice, you'll have the ability to treat respiratory diseases like bronchitis and asthma

Treat Psoriasis

With celery seeds nonetheless in tow, you can even treat skin diseases like psoriasis. Whether you take them in or blend them inside your juice, you'll take advantage of the nutrients and vitamins in these seeds.

Improve Blood Clotting Abilities

The vitamin K in celery plays a significant role in assisting your blood coagulum. With one glass of this vegetable, you'll consume 30% of the vitamin. For many individuals, celery acts as the natural cure from hair thinning to fat loss. Whatever you utilize this juice, you'll realize that you feel and appear far better after making celery and its juice a normal part of your diet.

Few studies have investigated medical ramifications of celery juice. However, celery does contain many essential nutrients that scientists consider as advantageous for people's health. Most research has concentrated on investigating the consequences of a number of the nutrients and antioxidants that this plant and its own seeds contain. Scientists think that these chemicals are advantageous in treating many health conditions.

Folks who are allergic or sensitive to celery should avoid eating this plant. Those who find themselves trying to lessen their sodium consumption ought to be conscious of total intake for the day from all foodstuffs, including celery. However, eating celery shouldn't cause problems for many people.

Not only is celery lower in calories, it also has several nutrients that are advantageous to the body. Celery helps to lower cholesterol levels and arthritis pain detoxifies the body, reduces high blood pressure and promotes the current health. They have demonstrated both antioxidant and anti-inflammatory activities that help to improve blood circulation pressure, regulate cholesterol levels and keep your heart healthy and strong.

Chapter 4

Green celery smoothie

Crunchy, crisp and refreshing, celery is a low-fat, low-calorie vegetable that may be eaten raw or cooked. Though it is a wholesome food choice, celery shouldn't be the central aspect of your daily diet, having a number of vegetables in your meal plan may be the key to healthy nutrition.

Among the great things about celery is that the vegetable is naturally saturated in dietary fiber. A 1-cup serving of diced celery contains 1.9 grams of fiber, based on the USDA. Celery is usually 95 percent water, additionally, it is lower in calories, providing only 19 in the same meal. While this merely provides 5 to 8 percent from the recommended intake of fibers, based on the National Academies of Sciences, it could cause complications for individuals who do not, as a rule, have a diet saturated in fiber.

A diet saturated in fiber has numerous health advantages, but an abrupt increase in fiber could cause digestive complications. If you're eating a whole lot of celery, you may experience constipation, gas or abdominal pain.

Celery can be high in insoluble fiber, which may cause pain in your digestive tract, particularly if you have an inflamed gut

Look out for Residual Pesticides

Based on the University of Washington Center for Ecogenetics & Environmental Health (CEEH), Celery is among the foods which have probably the most residual pesticides. Pesticides are known toxins, which, in sufficiently high quantities or with regular exposure, can result in toxicity in the heart and nervous system, as well as boost your risk for hormonal complications and cancer. Pesticides may also greatly increase your likelihood of skin, eye and lung irritation. Limit your consumption of conventionally grown celery to lessen your contact with harmful pesticides, or choose organic produce in order to avoid the bad ramifications of celery.

Add Variety

As an associate in the vegetable foods group and "other vegetables" subgroup, celery might help you meet up with the recommended intake of 2-3 cups of vegetables each day, as outlined inside the 2015-2020 Dietary Guidelines for Americans. You will need to eat a number of vegetables to obtain a balanced nutritional intake.

Add a daily mixture of beans and peas, leafy greens, starchy vegetables, and red and orange vegetables to be able to meet up with the Dietary Guidelines' full nutritional recommendation.

Avoid Possible Allergies

Based on the Anaphylaxis Campaign, celery allergy is rather common, especially in central Europe. People that have problems with pollen allergies may experience some allergic reactions when consuming celery.

Mild symptoms range between itching in the throat to more serious cases, where anaphylactic shock may result. Celery could cause an allergic attack whether it's cooked or raw. If you're worried about a potential allergy, consult a Health care professional to get tested.

Celery Seed Extract Effects

Celery supplements can be found as celery seed extract, fresh or dried seeds, tablets or as capsules filled with celery seed oil. Although celery seed and extract can be used to treat several health issues that few human studies support this but produces unwanted effects with its usage. Fresh celery contains important nutrients but celery seed extract in supplements could cause side effects.

Uses of Celery Seed

Celery is often consumed like a vegetable and its own components such as seeds are generally used as a food seasoning ingredient. Elements of the celery plant, botanically referred to as *Apium graveolens*, have already been used therapeutically for a large number of years. Ayurvedic medicine uses celery seed to take care of fluid retention, colds and flu, poor digestion, various kinds of arthritis and certain diseases on the liver and spleen.

An article in the 2013 Journal of Drug Discovery and Therapeutics reports that celery and celery seed tea tend to be used as a diuretic, this means it will help your body eliminate normal water by increasing urine output. Furthermore, potential celery seed benefits are the treatment of ailments such as edema, gout, flatulence, chronic pneumonia and obesity. Celery is an all-natural therapy for these along with other medical issues in animal studies but remains to become proven effective in humans.

A typical dietary herbal intervention for gout is celery. A report in, published in June 2018, investigated the result of celery and its own hydroalcoholic extracts on treating gout. Even though results demonstrated that celery could decrease the crystals level in mice, no human studies have been conducted. Even more, Invitro research is required to verify these preliminary findings.

Unwanted Effects from Celery Seeds

Although herbal treatments are usually accepted as complementary and alternative therapies in conjunction with additional medications, herbs can have unwanted effects and connect to various other herbs, supplements, and medications. Therefore, you should solely consider celery seed supplements under the supervision of physician.

Pregnant women shouldn't take celery supplements or drink celery seed tea. A written report in a Journal, released in Pharmacognosy Review in June 2017, says huge amounts of celery can lead to muscle contractions inside the uterus and uterine bleeding, both of which could raise the threat of miscarriage. The safety of taking celery oil and seeds if you're breastfeeding is unknown, so it is best to avoid usage during such period.

When you have low blood pressure, you need to take caution when contemplating celery seed extract being a supplement. Researches carried out in 2013, indicated that celery seed extract may decrease both systolic and diastolic blood pressure. Further studies had a need to confirm these results so, to try to take it out, monitor your blood circulation pressure if you're going for a celery supplement.

A number of the phenolic compounds in celery seeds could cause the skin to be very sensitive towards the sun's Ultraviolet rays. Do not make use of celery seed or apply celery seed oil if you're under the Sun for a long period of time. If you are using celery seed extract, be sure to employ sunscreen or sunblock lotions to safeguard your skin layer from sunburn.

Allergies to Celery

Celery may end up being dangerous for allergic individuals. It includes allergens that could provoke severe allergies, including anaphylaxis. According to Penn State University, if you're allergic to birch pollen, it's likely you'll also be allergic to celery seeds. There's cross-reactivity with all types of celery, including celery salt, celery root, celery seed and commercial products which contain celery seed, such as, Old Bay seasoning.

Symptoms of celery allergy can afflict the mouth area, with swelling and itching from the mouth, tongue and throat.

When the celery plant is infected by the fungus *Sclerotinia sclerotiorum*, skin contact could cause dermatitis in sensitive people. Additional reactions that may derive from handling the plant or eating huge amounts of celery seeds include tiredness, slowed breathing and decreased heartbeat.

An allergy to celery seed could cause rare but severe life-threatening reactions in a few people. In the event that you experience the following symptoms, get immediate medical assistance:

- A swollen throat or the constriction and tightening in the airways
- Shock, plus a severe drop in blood circulation pressure
- Rapid pulse
- Dizziness or lack of consciousness

Before going for a supplement containing celery seed extract, ask your physician if you're on any medication which could react to the herb. A few of these consist of lithium, diuretics, anticoagulants and thyroid medications.

Water & Celery Diet

The popularity of crash diets persists because these diets promise impossibly fast weight loss. Water and celery diet could be a low-calorie way to reduce a few pounds; however, eating only celery and drinking only water can leave your inside in a weakened nutritional state. Once you know the limitations of the fad diet, understand how you are able to reasonably contain both celery and drinking water in what you eat.

Water and celery diet has a minimal calorie that will help you drop weight.

Achieving Negative Calorie Balance

The low-calorie nature of celery, along with calorie-free water, places them within the group of "negative-calorie" foods, meaning you might burn up more calories digesting them than they actually contain. A researcher explains that attempting to lose weight by concentrating on possibly negative-calorie foods inhibits your capability to consume a balanced diet. Although, normal water is essential to your wellbeing, water gives the body no calories, vitamins or minerals.

Too Little Calories and Fats

As you slim down, you will need at least 1,200 calories to remain healthy if you're a female, and 1,600 calories if you're a Man, based on the National Institutes of Health. Eating 1,200 or 1,600 calories in celery alone, besides being unhealthy, will be almost impossible. To consume 1,200 calories or 1,600 calories, you'll need to take in 75 to 100 cups of raw celery each day. Celery offers exclusively a trace amount of fat, as 1 cup contains just 0.17 grams, and 100 cups contain 17 grams. The body needs fat to process nutrients and present your energy. Normal water contains no calories or fat.

Nutrients-free

A 1-cup serving of celery has significantly less than 1 grams of protein, 1.9 grams of natural sugar and 1.6 grams of fiber. When you need between 22 and 34 grams of fiber each day. In the event that you ate enough calories in celery to sustain you, you might consume around three to four occasions more dietary fiber than necessary. Celery also offers 40 milligrams of calcium per cup and 81 milligrams of sodium. If you're dieting, you might be restricting your sodium for the American Heart Association's 1,500-milligram recommendation. Eating celery the whole day could cause you to take in excessive amount of sodium.

Celery also includes 36 micrograms of folate, 3.1 milligrams of vitamin C and 453 International Units (IU) of vitamin A per cup. In the event that you try to eat 20 cups of celery, you'll consume 9,060 IU of vitamin A, far above the recommended levels of 3,000 IU for men and 2,310 IU for ladies. Excess vitamin A could be one factor in osteoporosis, based on the National Institutes of Health. While water is healthy, it offers the body with few vitamins or minerals.

Healthy Weight-Loss Strategies

Avoid using just celery and water while dieting, and instead incorporate the vitamin-rich vegetable inside your balanced weight-loss diet program, which adds a selection of foods from all of the food groups and enough calories to meet up your nutrient needs.

Add peanut butter to raw celery sticks for any snack with both healthy fats and protein; dip celery sticks in Greek yogurt blended with onions and herbs, and add celery to salads and soups. You are able to juice raw celery with apples and spinach for a wholesome drink. Water might help your bodyweight loss efforts, as normal water increases your feeling of fullness, which may assist you to control calorie consumption.

Detoxing with Celery Juice

Just like the water and celery diet, celery juice has even more hype than the fact. Based on the proponents with the celery juice detox, you need to drink 16 ounces of celery juice on an empty stomach first thing each day, which supposedly improves absorption and digestion. The celery juice testimonials declare that drinking the celery water improves energy, digestion, mood, and concentration. There is no medical evidence to aid these claims. Drinking celery juice, or any other kind of detox juice or diet, won't improve your natural detoxification system: your liver and kidneys. It's okay to drink celery juice occasionally, but it isn't a miracle cure as claimed.

Steps to making simple Celery Juice

Basically, fresh celery juice is among the most effective healing juices available to us. This clean, green drink may be the absolute best way to start out your day. Let this juice be an integral part of your day to day routine, and shortly you won't need to go each day without it!

Ingredients:

A couple of celery

Directions:

Rinse the celery and put it in a juicer. ***Drink immediately for the best results.***

Alternatively, you may chop the celery and blend it in a high-speed blender until smooth. Don't use water or ice for the best healing benefits, only use celery. Strain the blended celery well through an excellent mesh strainer, cheesecloth or nut milk bag and drink immediately.

Celery Juice Tips

If you wish to heal and improve your wellbeing quickly and efficiently, follow this program:

- Each morning, drink 16 ounces or even more of celery juice on a clear stomach. Make certain it's fresh, plain celery juice without additional ingredients. Celery juice is highly medicinal, not really a caloric drink, so you'll still need breakfast afterward to power you in the morning. Simply wait at least 15 to thirty minutes after drinking your celery juice before consuming other things.

- If you're sensitive and 16 ounces is an excessive amount, start with less and work the right path up. You can even drink much more than 16 ounces. Many people want to drink 32 ounces daily.

- Use organic celery whenever you can. If you're using conventional celery, make sure to wash it especially prior to juicing.

- If you discover the taste of the celery juice is too strong, you could juice one cucumber and/or one apple with the celery. While you get accustomed to it, increase the ratio of celery until your juice becomes only celery; the best benefits come when celery juice is consumed alone.

As you become accustomed to drinking this juice, feel free to raise the amount of celery or scale back on the other ingredients to make it even more celery if desired.

6 Reasons to love Celery Juice

- **It lowers inflammation**: Celery is packed with antioxidants, including quercetin, caffeic acid, and ferulic acid. Antioxidants are believed to combat free radical damage that plays a part in inflammation.

- **It supports fight against infections**: Celery continues to be utilized to fight infections for years after years because celery seed contains antimicrobial and antibacterial properties. It's also considered to prohibit bacterial growth and raise the immune system.

- **It may help prevent liver disease**: Since celery has diuretic properties, it's considered to support, flush poisons from your body and promote liver and kidney health.

- **It may support lower cholesterol and high blood pressure**: Celery contains a distinctive compound called 3-n-butylphthalide (BuPh), which has been proven in studies (using celery seed extract like a supplement) to lessen overall cholesterol and help with hypertension.

- **It could reduce bloating and urinary system infections):** Celery has a diuretic influence on your body, which eliminates fluid retention and may help boost digestion which can result in less bloating. Since it decreases the crystals and boosts urine production, in addition, it can help prevent urinary system infections.

Steps to make Celery-Ginger Juice

To make celery juice, all you have to use is a juicer or high-speed blender. but in the event that you don't have a Juicer, use your blender instead. Run one or two bunches of celery stalks with the juicer that may extract the fiber and leave you with just the juice! It was discovered that a 2-pack of celery stalks makes about 16 ounces of juice.

Blend the celery until it appears like a smoothie. You can include a splash of water if needed, but it's likely best to use only a small amount of liquid as possible, so you don't dilute the juice. (A high-speed blender like Vitamix can blend veggies without added water- just utilize the tamper.) Pour the pureed celery juice right into a nut-milk bag to strain out the pulp, then drink the juice which you squeezed out!

Preserving Celery Juice In advance

It is strongly recommended that you drink fresh vegetable juice once you make it, but if you're in a rush in the mornings, you may make it a day beforehand and put it inside a tightly sealed mason jar inside the fridge. If you are using a masticating juicer, like my Omega juicer, your juice should last for 3 days. (You should take advantage of Omega juicer if you have, for juicing celery stalks, given that they easily fit into the chute, but you shouldn't utilize it for additional items since it takes too much time to chop everything into skinny pieces.)

Unwanted Effects of Celery Juice

Below are a few unwanted effects that people might experience:

- **A dancing stomach**

It is heard that celery juice can enhance digestion by increasing the hydrochloric acid in your stomach. (If you've been pregnant before, it literally feels like a baby kick.)

- **A laxative effect**

In the event that constipation tends to happen, this might help. Saltwater is known as a laxative, and since celery is usually packed with natural salts and is incredibly hydrating, we could simply assume that's why it had an almost-immediate laxative effect in you after drinking it.

Besides that, the various other side effects that you'll experience will all be positive, you'll feel less bloated and have less cravings for sweets, therefore you can't complain. You'll definitely feel great after trying this out.

Celery-ginger juice recipe

This celery juice recipe tastes amazing, especially because of the addition of cucumber, ginger, lemon, and green apple. *It forms the low-sugar drink that kick-starts your morning.*

Prep Time: Five minutes

Total Time: Five minutes

Servings: 1

Ingredients:

- 1 small bunch celery
- 1/2 cucumber
- 1 large green apple
- 1/2 lemon
- 1 -inch knob of ginger

Instruction:

In case your juicer includes a "high" and "low" setting, run the celery and cucumber first through the reduced setting. Then switch it to high and run the apple, lemon and ginger from the juicer. You can try to sandwich the little bit of ginger between your apple and lemon such that it stays put and is simpler to juice.

Drink the juice immediately, or preserve it in an airtight mason jar for 24 hours inside the fridge.

Chapter 5

Most asked questions on celery juice

What is the perfect amount of celery juice to get the healing benefits?

16 ounces of straight celery juice each day is fantastic for getting its healing benefits. Upping your intake as much as 24 to 32 ounces each day can be hugely good for anyone battling with chronic illness or symptoms.

Just how much celery is required to produce 16 oz of juice?

One large bunch typically makes 16 oz of juice.

When is the best time to drink celery juice?

The optimum time to drink celery juice is each day on a clear stomach before you consume other things apart from water or lemon water (wait for at least 15 to thirty minutes after the lemon before having your celery juice). Celery juice is really medicinal, not really a caloric drink, so you'll still need breakfast afterward to power you in the morning. Simply wait at least 15 to thirty minutes after drinking your celery juice before consuming other things.

If you're struggling to consume your celery juice first thing each day before food, then your second-best option would be to drink it 15 to 30 minutes before eating something or 30 to 60 minutes after eating a little snack or 2 hours after eating a heavier meal anytime throughout the day. If you're having 32 ounces per day, you may want it in two 16-ounce portions. You are able to drink the first serving each day on an empty stomach before eating and the next in the late afternoon or early evening, at least 15 to thirty minutes before consuming the next meal.

Which juicer would you recommend?

Masticating juicers will be the best juicers to make celery juice. Omega Juicers are excellent depending on your finances, but any juicer will still work.

Does the celery need to be organic?

Organic is most beneficial, but in the event that you can't get organic don't worry. You can buy conventionally grown celery. Then wash each stalk having a drop of natural fragrance-free dish soap, accompanied by rinsing in water. In the event that you don't possess natural clear dish soap, supply the celery an instant rinse in tepid to warm water. Ensuring to rinse each stalk.

Can I get celery juice in advance?

It's better to drink celery juice soon after juicing. But in the event that you don't have another option, don't let it proceed past 1 day (a day). If using this program, be sure to seal it inside a mason jar, and store within the refrigerator.

Could it be okay to include lime or lemon to my celery juice?

Celery juice is most effective on its own. Adding other ingredients to the juice will dilute its medicinal houses. This consists of lemon, lime, ginger, apple, orange, leafy greens, carrot, beet, or any other ingredient. Wait 15-30 minutes after drinking your celery juice, before consuming other things.

Are there other things that can be put into celery juice to make it more helpful?

Celery juice is actually a healing tool for the chronically ill. They have healed and are constantly healing thousands of people worldwide. Sadly, a lot of people are now wanting to make use of the popularity of celery juice by changing the recipe and adding new ingredients to allow them to call it their own, and benefit from it. They recommend adding ingredients like collagen, apple cider vinegar, and activated charcoal to celery juice, but these three products all destroy and denature celery juice when put into it, removing most of its original healing properties and bringing ingredients into the body that don't support healing.

For the protection of your health, it's important you know about how misleading and unhelpful these trends that compromise the purity and power of celery juice are. These trends have already been started by people who don't actually have confidence in celery juice as well as the healing properties it possesses. They never knew of its existence like a healing tool before the global celery juice movement, we started to organically reach thousands of people because it is indeed effective at assisting to heal all sorts of health symptoms and conditions.

These financial investor who are trendsetters don't even understand what it is about celery juice that makes it so effective, such as for example, its undiscovered sodium cluster salts that destroy the cell membranes of pathogens and allow them to be killed off and the way the cluster salts rebuild hydrochloric acid. Without focusing on how celery juice works and just why, they can't learn how to consume it to get its benefits and exactly how vital it really is not to bring ingredients such as collagen, apple cider vinegar and, and activated charcoal into it.

Knowing the proper way to drink celery juice is crucial to get its benefits. There are a few nutritional compounds that will help activate or improve the healing properties of celery juice a lot more. Some of these nutritional compounds include magnesium, l-glutamine, and choline for instance.

Can I simply eat celery rather than juicing it?

The reason why we juice the celery versus consuming it is basically because juicing and removing the pulp (fiber) may be the only way to obtain the powerful healing benefits for healing chronic illness. There's a style that is now happening that recommends leaving the pulp inside the drink and encourages blended celery versus celery juice, which removes the fiber. Do not be misled by this trend. Leaving the pulp in could keep you from receiving the initial healing and the great things about celery juice.

Consuming celery itself is effective and should participate in your diet, but you'll not have the ability to consume enough celery to acquire the advantages of juicing it. You wouldn't have the ability to have the concentrated undiscovered cluster salts, that all the following will do:

- Promptly rebuild your hydrochloric acid, which means that, your stomach can breakdown protein. If protein isn't divided properly it'll cause gut rot. Strong hydrochloric acid is vital that you kill off pathogens entering the mouth area.

- Celery Juice increases and strengthens your bile. Strong bile is very important to the breakdown of fats, as well as for the killing off pathogens; which have made their way into the body. Ingesting straight celery wouldn't enable you to receive enough of celery's cluster salts; which acts as antiseptics for pathogens.
- Celery juice restores your central nervous system. Removes old toxins and poisons, such as for example old pharmaceuticals from your own liver.

Is celery juice okay to take while pregnant?

Yes, celery juice is safe and healthy to take while pregnant. When you have any concerns, you are able to check with your doctor.

Can breastfeeding women drink celery juice?

Celery juice is incredible for breastfeeding. It could offer an abundance of trace minerals, vitamin C and neurotransmitter chemicals like the undiscovered sodium cluster salts for the infant to build up healthy, strong organs. Celery juice also helps clean and detoxify the breast milk, purifying it therefore the baby receives the purest breast milk possible.

Can babies and children drink celery juice?

Yes, celery juice is incredible for the medical and development of babies and children.

Could it be normal to see a big change in bowel motions after drinking celery juice?

Some individuals may experience an alteration in their bowel motions when they begin to consume celery juice. That is a standard detox reaction that a lot of people that have a higher degree of toxins may experience. Celery juice will kill off unproductive bacteria within the gut and can also help purge the liver. This may bring about loose stools as your body pushes out the toxins from an extremely toxic liver. Everyone today possess some extent of liver toxicity, which can result in countless symptoms and conditions. The loose stools will pass as the body heals and you'll notice your bowel motions become more standard and healthier than ever before. If you discover celery juice is too cleansing, try 16 oz of straight cucumber juice. Cucumber juice doesn't have the same benefits celery juice has, nonetheless it is quite gentle and a fantastic choice until you can restart celery juice.

Am I going to experience a rise in symptoms after drinking celery juice?

Celery juice is quite healing, and the undiscovered sodium cluster salts will quickly kill off pathogens like viruses such as Epstein-Barr and Shingles, as well as bacteria such as Streptococcus in the body immediately. For some, if they've already experienced some symptoms on/off in their life such as fatigue or other symptoms, it's possible that in some instances, these folks may temporarily experience the symptoms again. These symptoms are going to be short and brief as your body heals and cleans up. That is a robust healing step that celery juice can provide for long-term health without symptoms.

However, often when someone reports feeling a rise in symptoms and thinks it's due to the celery juice, it'll actually be due to another thing happening within their body, life or diet, however, the celery juice unfairly takes the blame. It's vital that you know very well what else could possibly be happening in the body and exactly how dietary choices along with other lifestyle factors could possibly be resulting in the upsurge in symptoms and conditions someone could possibly be experiencing and how exactly to properly support your body to heal. It's never been more critical to empower you to ultimately become a specialist on the real factors behind your symptoms and conditions.

Could it be normal to get bloated after drinking celery juice?

Celery juice rapidly boosts digestion. It can do this by prompting the liver to improve bile production and instantly strengthening the stomach's hydrochloric acid production. Which in turn begins to breakdown old undigested rotting protein, old rancid fats trapped in the bottom from the stomach, and in the tiny intestinal tract which has been there for many years in everyone. Once these fats and proteins dissolve, bloating will go away for nearly everyone who's coping with chronic bloating issues.

But also, for some, a sense of bloating may appear that may be mild to severe, based on how toxic someone's digestive system is becoming and just how much old rotten

73

undigested debris is within their digestive system. As they continue to use celery juice the correct way long-term, the problem and toxicity of the digestive system will improve and bloating can disappear so long as their additional ingesting choices are within the rules of a healthy clean diet.

Does celery juice contain oxalates?

There's a myth that leafy vegetables or herbs like celery are saturated in oxalates and so are therefore harmful. That is completely incorrect and it is preventing many folks from obtaining some powerful and needed nutrients and healing properties supplied by foods considered to become saturated in oxalates. Oxalates aren't the concern they may be thought to be.

You will find oxalates in almost every single fruit and vegetable on earth. The vast selection of nutrients in so-called high oxalate leafy greens and celery are a few of the most nutritious open to us. Medical research and science haven't discovered that you will find anti-oxalates in fruits, vegetables, and leafy greens that avoid the oxalates from causing us the damage the existing trend tells us they are causing. In reality, these food types don't cause us any harm, rather they offer us critical healing nutrients like phytochemicals, vitamins, and minerals.

May I consider celery juice powder or celery powder rather than drinking fresh celery juice?

No, celery powder and celery juice powder can't replace fresh celery juice. Celery juice powder and celery powder don't offer the benefits that 16 ounces of fresh straight celery juice can. Selling celery juice powders and putting celery inside supplements will turn into a popular trend as celery juice becomes a lot more well known and folks make an effort to profit from the global celery juice trend that is healing the chronically ill. Stay away from many of these fads. They certainly are a waste of money plus they don't provide same healing benefits as drinking straight, fresh celery juice each day.

Are there nitrates in celery juice?

Celery and celery juice can't contain any nitrates which are activated or harmful unless the celery has oxidized or has been dehydrated. The naturally occurring nitrates in celery don't exist once the celery or fresh celery juice hasn't yet oxidized. When fresh celery juice or celery does oxidize, exactly like when any herb, vegetable or fruit oxidizes, a naturally occurring nitrate can form. But this naturally occurring nitrate can be never harmful at all, shape or form. Celery juice powder and celery powder have oxidized to allow them to contain naturally occurring nitrates because that developed from the oxidation process.

These nitrates won't be the same selection of nitrates which are believed to get irritating for some people. It's vital that you realize that not absolutely all nitrates will be the same, exactly like everyone is not similar, all water aren't exactly the same, all sugar aren't similar, and every protein isn't exactly the same. For instance, gluten can be an entirely different protein compared to the protein inside meat or the protein inside nuts. Also, the naturally occurring nitrates that may develop within an oxidized type of celery such as celery powder, and celery juice powder won't be the same as the harmful nitrates which can be put into the meat and all sorts of other products.

Also, *nitrates* will vary to *nitrites*; they're not a similar thing. Even celery powder, which does contain naturally occurring nitrates, can't be relied upon as a way for treating foods such as pickles or meat since it nonetheless doesn't contain nitrites. Fresh celery juice also doesn't contain nitrites. Anything naturally occurring in celery and celery juice isn't harmful. This is actually the same for pure celery powder and pure celery juice powder. However, harmful nitrates could be put into celery powder or celery juice powder by the business that means it is or uses it in another product. Your fresh celery juice cannot feature harmful nitrates in it if you don't include them in yourself.

In the event that you don't drink fresh celery juice because you think it includes harmful nitrates, you then are unfortunately likely to lose the initial healing opportunity fresh celery juice, which will not contain nitrates, can offer.

Just how long does it take to get the advantages of drinking celery juice?

This will depend on what condition the individual is in. Everyone feels great things about some kind within their 1st week of drinking celery juice in the proper amount and correctly regularly. Many people even feel benefited after their first juice. Everything depends on the individual and their conditions, such as their health issues and symptoms, how toxic and overburdened their liver has been, different pathogens and poisons such as pesticides, solvents, herbicides, toxic heavy metals, and all sorts of various chemicals and toxins. If someone is coping with weight issues, if indeed they have a whole lot of putrefied and rancid fats within their colon, and/or a whole lot of bacteria within their intestinal tract such as *Streptococcus*, this may also affect the healing timeline.

The quantity of stress someone is experiencing within their life, what else they choose to consume and drink furthermore with their straight celery juice, and their other way of life habits may also be likely involved in just how long it requires for them to definitely feel the huge benefits, however, a lot of people do experience a difference quickly. Some people who've been drinking celery juice for a long period get accustomed to how sound or just how much better it makes them than if they weren't drinking it. They quit drinking celery juice temporarily, like many do, and discover they don't think nearly as good anymore. They understand at this time precisely how instrumental the celery juice was in assisting them come to feel better.

It's vital that you know that even though someone doesn't see or look at the advantages of drinking celery juice quickly, it doesn't mean the huge benefits aren't happening. Everybody who drinks celery juice receives benefits immediately, as the healing powers of celery juice begin working immediately upon entering your body. For a lot, normally it takes a little bit of time to discover or feel the benefits within a tangible way they are able to notice, despite the fact that the celery juice continues to be providing healing advantages from the initial drink internally.

Will there be an excessive amount of sodium in celery juice?

All salt isn't similar, exactly like all sugar isn't exactly the same. Consuming high fructose corn syrup, which is detrimental to health, isn't exactly like consuming an apple, that may bring healing for the liver and offer an abundance of critical nutrients. So, don't get confused by the theory that salt may be the same because it's not.

In the event that you hear someone say that there's an excessive amount of salt in celery juice, they're not correct. The sodium cluster groups in celery juice certainly are a subgroup of sodium. Science and research may not even found out all of the variations of trace minerals and subgroups of sodium that have a home in celery juice. Sodium cluster salts are healing for your body and we can't have enough of these. Sixteen ounces of celery juice on a regular basis provides these sodium cluster salts we so greatly need.

Celtic sea salt or Himalayan rock salt are entirely different types of sodium. Regardless of how top-quality the salt, putting Celtic sea salt or Himalayan rock salt in a glass or two or on your own food isn't exactly like consuming enough of the undiscovered sodium cluster salts from celery juice. Sodium cluster salts will be the only type of sodium that destroys pathogens, helps detox your body and help restore electrolytes and neurotransmitter chemicals. The sodium in celery juice can be medicinal sodium that's designed for your bloodstream as well as your body whereas you will need to be careful of consuming an excessive amount of the sort of sodium that will come in, even the best quality salts.

May I juice celery root rather than celery?

No, celery root is often a different plant towards the large bunches of celery stalks with leaves. Juicing celery root won't but supply the same healing benefits.

Toxins in Celery

Celery contains toxins called psoralens with potentially carcinogenic effects and goitrogens with potentially anti-thyroid effects. Celery can be among the vegetables highest in pesticide content unless it really is organically grown, and it is vulnerable to some sort of mold called mycotoxins. You will find, however, methods to grow, select, prepare and consume celery to reduce the associated health threats. Celery contains particular waste, including one with carcinogenic properties.

Psoralens

Celery contains some sort of natural toxin called psoralens that may cause your skin to become even more sensitive towards the harmful ramifications of ultraviolet radiation, a disorder referred to as Phytophotodermatitis, therefore, they are believed to be photocarcinogenic. According to David H. Watson in his publication "Natural Toxicants in Food;" cooking, and especially boiling, reduces the psoralens in celery and will not destroy them completely. Ramifications of phytophotodermatitis consist of skin rashes and discolorations, blisters and sunburn.

Goitrogens

Also called glucosinolates, goitrogens certainly are a compound manufactured from sugar and sulfur that may have a poor influence on the thyroid, specifically inhibiting its iodine uptake. According to a report titled "The Nutritional Need for Naturally Occurring Toxins in Plant Foodstuffs" cited within the FDA Poisonous Plants Database, goitrogens in vegetables like celery are estimated to take into account 4 percent of goiter incidences, or swelling from the thyroid, inside the world's population.

Pesticides

According to a written report released in 2010 by the general public non-profit health group, inorganic celery reaches the top in the "Dirty Dozen" set of fruits & vegetables containing probably the most pesticides, with 64 types of pesticide in each serving. Because celery does not have any protective skin to soak up harmful pesticides, individuals are much more likely to ingest those pesticides when eating the vegetable. Chronic ramifications of residual pesticides in food on human health continue to be a topic of many studies. Pesticides in food have already been linked to specific immune dysfunctions and cancers. Additional evidence has linked food pesticides to neurological and developmental problems in children, including ADHD.

Nitrates

Celery is saturated in nitrates, which, when subjected to certain micro-organisms within foods and in the gastrointestinal tract, could be reduced to potentially toxic nitrites. In large enough doses, nitrites could cause Methemoglobinemia, or the increased loss of haemoglobin's oxygen-carrying ability, as well as death. However, evidence has only linked high nitrate vegetable sources to nitrite toxicity in infants.

Mycotoxins

Celery is susceptible to certain molds called mycotoxins, including aflatoxin or black mold. Aflatoxins are known as carcinogens. Other potential health ramifications of mycotoxin consumption include abdominal pain, vomiting, edema, convulsions, liver damage, mental impairment and issues with digesting, absorbing and metabolizing food.

The psoralens in celery result from a brownish fungus referred to as pink rot. Just eat celery without brown spots in order to avoid consuming psoralens. Avoid consuming the pesticide inorganic celery by purchasing just organic celery or from an area grower you trust. Its insufficient skin makes washing any pesticides from the celery extremely difficult.

Amount of Celery Juice to Drink

Drinking 16 ounces of pure celery juice on a clear stomach daily can offer you with a large number of health advantages. But, if you're a newbie to celery juice, work the right path up from 4-8 ounces though, as you may experience severe die-off symptoms if the body is actually toxic. You are able to drink far more, but it should not exceed 10 glasses.

How to Drink the Juice Correctly

- Drink 16 ounces (2 glasses) of pure celery juice each morning on an empty stomach.
- Wait for 20-30 minutes before you consume other things, drink or food.
- Don't eat any fatty foods, i.e. nuts, seeds, avocado, olives at least 2 hours after consuming celery juice. Also, make an effort to cut down your current fat consumption.
- Use organic celery whenever you can. In case you have conventional celery, be sure to wash every stalk thoroughly with non-scented soap.
- Be sure never to mix anything into the celery juice, not stevia or other sweeteners, water, lemon juice, apple cider vinegar nor other fruit or vegetable juices.
- Don't drink it in the center of your day when you've already consumed other foodstuffs and drinks.

- Drink freshly made celery juice. It ought to be consumed within a day of juicing it (store in a sealed jar in fridge). Remember that the juice loses its potency by hour.
- Celery powder, celery juice powder, and celery tablets won't replace fresh juice. The medicinal cluster salts in celery juice are suspended in a full-time solution and cannot stay alive outside newly juiced celery. The powerful enzymes in celery juice may also be ruined along the way of fabricating a tablet or powder. Also, eating celery won't provide you with the same benefits.

Common Mistakes people make

- Consuming celery juice with food.
- Mixing other things with their celery juice, e.g. sweeteners, drinking water, lime or lemon juice, ginger, collagen, protein powders, etc.
- Consuming a high-fat diet, especially eating high-fat foods after consuming celery juice.
- Not drinking enough celery juice.

- Preparing the juice in big batches - for some couple of days in advance.
- Buying pasteurized celery juice.
- Ingesting unproductive foods, e.g. gluten, eggs, dairy, corn, soy, pork.
- Not being consistent and quitting after a week or so.
- Some individuals feel the huge benefits already after a couple of hours, but also for some it could even take up to a year to notice major difference.

Chapter 6

Testimonials

Anonymous

"I've seen an enormous improvement in my own digestion, once I consume celery juice on an empty stomach first thing each day. When I initially started with celery juice, I saw plenty of impurities come to the top of my skin, meaning, most of the poisons had been being purged from the inside out. It had been very difficult never to pick within my skin (can anyone relate?) but after 14 days of my celery juice routine my skin was glowing! I likewise have seen a rise in my vigor a lot in order that I don't possess any cravings for coffee which is nearly just a little annoying because I really like producing my lattes now I move my latte ritual towards the afternoon."

Ciara jones

"The celery juice trend gets a whole lot of flack within the media. It's being deemed like a "fad" that "really does not have any benefits beyond hydration" and honestly it makes me sad to find out as the media absolutely loves knocking things it doesn't understand. It makes me sad as the deep healing celery juice provides is next level, and one which should at least get an opportunity (many people are different obviously)."

Victoria Loius

"I usually do have pollen driven headaches each day for about a week. Once I started juicing, I really was amazed to find out those headaches disappear from day 1! Plus they never have returned either.

Secondly, after about 5 days of juicing, I tried to go without rinsing my nose at night. Also to my wonderful surprise I could sleep quite nicely. When my supply was off and I went without juicing for approximately 5 days, I also resumed rinsing. However, when I re-established my celery juice routine, I also quit rinsing and haven't had the necessity for it since that time.

Another positive thing I noticed was the elimination. I wasn't constipating like before, but this was a complete fresh level . For 3-4 days I visited toilet three times a day, After all properly! Once I had been completely empty, it returned to normal. I assume it'll take a lot longer to determine results using the nails and fibroids, so I'll just continue heading."

Sonia larry

"The very next day I went for celery and started juicing. I had developed a "fairly healthy" diet plan before I started celery juicing but was convinced I had a lot of contaminants to dump, therefore I started small - 2 oz. Then, I built it up every day till I drank 16 ounces each day first thing each day before I fashioned anything else to consume or drink.

Danny lewis

"I have already been celery juicing for just one month now as well as the benefits up to now is vigor and elimination. However, my suggestion is usually to start out slow, since it can be hugely bloating initially. Celery juice is fairly filling and I usually get a "clean" cold rush to my stomach after I drink it. This feeling sticks beside me until I consume solid foods thirty minutes later."

Paul dreig

"Who knew I'd end up having a direct romance with celery juice. There have been jus 3 bunches left on the shelves since there is a legit celery shortage. I've been drinking celery juice for six months now and also have noticed such a notable difference in my own morning energy, especially given that my placenta pills have died. My skin glows, my gut health is on point, my postpartum inflammation has truly gone down enormously and my experience was so damn good."

Melinda Iyke

"These are the huge benefits I've experienced from consistently drinking celery juice each day:

- My skin feels more hydrated and smooth
- Personally, I become less hungry

- Personally, I become more nourished
- My sight became better

We don't experience occasional bloating anymore

Personally, I feel overall great after I drink celery juice. However, buying green juice is expensive, making it too complicated (you must have a refrigerator stocked with greens). Together with it, I don't enjoy drinking green juice without adding fruit for sweetness, while celery juice tastes just fine alone."

rosewood

"I actually started juicing straight celery juice after hearing about any of it a couple of weeks ago and I'll never return! ONCE I drink it I have a great deal of strength, like wire, however in a great way 😊 and undoubtedly it CLEANS you out! My skin is cleaner since starting, my digestion is way better, minimal bloating whereas before I had been constantly bloated, it took away my craving for coffee, I literally stopped cold turkey and didn't have any side-effects and I've been drinking coffee for nearly twenty years 😁. My brain fog disappeared on day 2 and hasn't returned, my thinking is superior whereas before it had been so foggy. I hate celery, to have, but I'll never stop drinking it very first thing each day, they have literally changed my entire life. One bulk in my own juicer each morning"

Chris Uther

"I could personally attest to celery juice and precisely how well it can benefit from IBS. I've been coping with IBS-C flareups for days gone by three years which leaves me bloated, lethargic, and constipated. I've attempted a countless amount of things both prescribed and natural but nothing has helped me just as much as drinking celery juice daily.I started drinking celery juice after hearing just how much it had helped my best friend's grandfather with a few of his ailments and seeing everything over my Instagram feed.

After drinking it first thing each day for weekly I used to be hooked. In a few days, my stomach was considerably less bloated, I felt like I had developed even more sustained energy, and I was a lot more regular. I'll admit, the taste from the juice was a bit much when I started drinking it in the beginning but I now find myself craving it inside the mornings! Celery juice is a wonderful addition to my morning ritual, also to my health overall."

Larry Fred

"My spouse and I started doing celery juice two months ago, the very first thing within the AM on a clear stomach, and it's the thing that appears to be helping my migraines. I had 10-12 migraines per month and during the last 3 years I've attempted everything (eastern and western) and nothing spent some time working which means this seems such as a miracle."

Will R. Smith

"I just juiced celery for thirty days straight to find out if there is validity behind each one of these health claims. The primary benefit I wanted was to ease my psoriasis, that I had heard celery juice may help treat. I've psoriasis on my scalp, and it's been something I have already been coping with for eight years. I couldn't find anything to greatly help address it because Personally, I stay away from putting chemicals, or anything unnatural, into my own body. This implies I refused to consider steroids or toxic skin medications that my doctor suggested.

I likewise have been fighting gut and hormone issues and also have been dealing with a naturopath to heal. So, I had been also seeking to increase my gut health insurance and rebalance my hormones through drinking celery juice.

It's vital that you note that of these 30 days, I did not change anything in my own diet beyond juicing celery. I also made a decision to ease my way with it by starting with 8 ounces for the first couple of days before investing in 16 ounces every day.

Juicing celery almost every other day was far more realistic for my entire life. This way, I possibly could nonetheless ensure I'm used to be drinking in a 24-hour period. I generally would juice two days' worth at the same time, then drink 16 ounces immediately and save the other 16 ounces for another morning."

Miemie Thienry

"The most immediate effect I see is on digestion, you certainly spot the flow! And I could attest that it's most likely ideal for removing toxins as my skin looks much clearer and brighter when on a regular basis! I have already been drinking it first thing each day, after my lemon drinking water, for almost 12 months now (aside from days when I must dash to work at 6 am. I really like it!"

Nuella Gaby

"My first couple of days of drinking celery juice, I felt absolutely amazing. My digestion was great, my bloating was heading down and I felt a lot more vigor but after 4-6 hits, my bloating returned (it actually worsened), and I was completely supported. I continued to juice regardless and I am so glad I did so, because after those couple of days passed, my digestion, bloating and psoriasis became much better than in the past. My psoriasis didn't completely disappear, nonetheless it continues to be drastically alleviated.

I have decided to continue to drink celery juice each morning. Yes, it's time-consuming to get ready, however, the effect it has on my health makes it a lot more than worthwhile.

Winifred Kins

"The discomforts of indigestion, bloating, as well as acid reflux in many cases are due to low gastric acid. Studies show that folks with Hashimoto's (the autoimmune thyroid condition) and hypothyroidism (low thyroid) frequently have low, or insufficient gastric acid, and low gastric acid which causes a wheel of undesirable health consequences. Most of us are too acquainted with the fact that whenever we are stressed among the first what to walk out whack could be our digestion. That's where the superhero of celery juice steps in, as its natural sodium content, raises gastric acid, so when taken, the very first thing each day primes you for is easy digestion for all of those other days. Gastric acid is vital for the digestion of food, particularly protein. In case your stomach acid can be lowered, your body then must play a vital role as an asset to attempt to digest that food, thus, causing you to be tired. This also results in liver backlog, so there's less chance your liver can match the onslaught of waste it must proceed from mere everyday living, as well as its job of balancing blood sugar levels and recycling and producing new hormones among its many other tasks.

The liver is really a heavy-duty organ-and as you can plainly see, that's where the cycle continues, continually overwhelming your body so that it never includes a chance to reset, heal, and thrive. Occasionally, this can be Okay (most of us get stressed every once in a while!), but if that is happening continually, it could lead to considerably more chronic and serious manifestations of disease in the torso. Once I started drinking celery juice, I pointed out that my food digested easier. Rather than uncomfortable feelings of fullness and heaviness after meals, I instead felt satiated but nonetheless light and continue on with my activities very easily."